DEALING WITH HEARTBURN DURING PREGNANCY

A comprehensive guide to heartburn and acid reflux relief through every trimester

Dr Stacy Hills

Table of Contents

HOW TO USE THIS BOOK

Welcome to your comprehensive guide on managing heartburn during pregnancy. This book is designed to be your trusted companion, offering practical advice, medical insights, and personal stories to help you navigate this aspect of your pregnancy journey. To get the most out of this book, here are some guidelines and tips to help you along the way:

Start with the Basics

Begin by reading the Introduction. This section will provide you with a foundational understanding of heartburn during pregnancy, why it occurs, and the importance of managing it effectively. This context will help you appreciate the subsequent chapters and how they build upon this knowledge.

Tailor Your Reading to Your Needs

This book is structured to be both comprehensive and flexible. Each chapter addresses a specific aspect of heartburn management, allowing you to focus on the topics most relevant to your situation. If you're experiencing severe heartburn, you might want to jump directly to the chapter on dealing with severe heartburn. If you're interested in natural remedies, the section on holistic and alternative approaches will be particularly useful.

Utilize the Glossary

Medical and technical terms can sometimes be confusing. Use the Glossary of Terms in the Appendices section to familiarize yourself with any unfamiliar terminology. This quick reference guide will help you better understand the information presented throughout the book.

Engage with the Dietary Charts and Meal Plans

Diet plays a crucial role in managing heartburn. The dietary charts and meal plans provided in the Appendices offer practical guidance on what to eat and what to avoid. These resources are designed to be easy to follow and can be adapted to your personal preferences and dietary needs. Try incorporating these meal plans into your daily routine to see which foods work best for you.

Incorporate Exercises and Yoga Poses

Regular physical activity can significantly impact your well-being and help manage heartburn. The sample exercises and yoga poses provided in the Appendices are designed to be safe and beneficial for pregnant women. Even if you're new to exercise or yoga, these gentle routines are a great way to stay active and reduce stress.

Always listen to your body and modify poses as needed to ensure comfort and safety.

Take Notes and Reflect

As you read through each chapter, take notes on the strategies and tips that resonate with you. Reflect on how you can incorporate these suggestions into your daily life. Keeping a journal of your experiences can also be helpful, allowing you to track what works and what doesn't, and to discuss your findings with your healthcare provider.

Consult Your Healthcare Provider

While this book offers a wealth of information and practical advice, it's essential to consult with your healthcare provider before making any significant changes to your diet, exercise routine, or treatment plan. Your provider can offer personalized guidance and ensure that any new practices are safe for you and your baby.

Engage with Personal Stories

The personal stories and experiences shared in this book are meant to inspire and reassure you. Reading about other mothers who have successfully managed heartburn can provide valuable insights and emotional support. These stories highlight that you're not alone in your journey, and that effective strategies do exist.

Explore Additional Resources

The Resources and Support section at the end of the book offers further reading, support groups, and contact information for healthcare professionals. These resources are invaluable if you need more in-depth information or additional support. Don't hesitate to reach out to these communities and professionals for guidance and encouragement.

Frequently Asked Questions

The Frequently Asked Questions chapter is a handy resource for quick answers to common concerns about heartburn during pregnancy. Whether you're looking for immediate relief tips or long-term management strategies, this section provides concise and practical advice. Refer to this chapter whenever you need a quick refresher or immediate guidance.

Stay Positive and Patient

Managing heartburn during pregnancy can be challenging, but remember that you are doing an incredible job. Stay positive, be patient with yourself, and celebrate the small victories along the way. Each step you take towards managing your heartburn is a step towards a healthier, more comfortable pregnancy.

Connect with the Content

This book is designed to be engaging and relatable. As you read, imagine you're having a conversation with a friend who understands what you're going through. Feel free to highlight passages, bookmark sections, and revisit chapters as needed. This book is here to support you, so make it your own.

Feedback and Reflection

Your journey through pregnancy is unique, and your feedback is invaluable. Reflect on how the strategies and advice in this book have impacted your experience. What worked well for you? What challenges did you face? Your insights can help other expectant mothers who are navigating similar challenges.

In conclusion, this book is a comprehensive resource designed to support you in managing heartburn during pregnancy. By following these guidelines and engaging with the content, you can make the most out of this book and find effective strategies to improve your comfort and well-being. Thank you for allowing me to be a part of your journey. Wishing you a healthy, happy, and heartburn-free pregnancy!

INTRODUCTION

As a mother-to-be, you're likely navigating a whirlwind of emotions, experiences, and changes. Pregnancy is a miraculous journey, a time when your body transforms to nurture the tiny life growing within you. It's a period filled with anticipation, joy, and sometimes a few discomforts, such as heartburn. If you're experiencing this burning sensation in your chest, you're not alone. Heartburn is a common companion during pregnancy, but it doesn't have to overshadow this beautiful journey.

Heartburn during pregnancy is not just an annoyance; it can significantly impact your daily life and overall well-being. Understanding why heartburn occurs and how to manage it effectively can make a world of difference. During pregnancy, your body undergoes numerous changes, both hormonal and physical, that can contribute to heartburn. The hormone progesterone, which helps relax the muscles of your uterus to accommodate your growing baby, also relaxes the valve that separates your esophagus from your stomach. This relaxation allows stomach acid to flow back up into the esophagus, causing that familiar burning sensation. Additionally, as your baby grows, the increasing size of your uterus puts pressure on your stomach, which can also lead to acid reflux.

Managing heartburn is crucial not only for your comfort but also for maintaining your overall health and well-being during pregnancy. Persistent heartburn can lead to complications such as esophagitis, a condition where the oesophagus becomes inflamed. This can result in difficulty swallowing, chest pain, and even bleeding. Furthermore, chronic heartburn can affect your sleep, appetite, and mood, leading to fatigue and stress, which are the last things you need during this crucial time.

That's where this book comes in. My goal is to provide you with a comprehensive guide to understanding and managing heartburn during pregnancy. This book is designed to be your go-to resource, offering practical advice, medical insights, and personal stories to help you navigate this aspect of your pregnancy journey. We'll explore the causes and symptoms of heartburn, delve into dietary and lifestyle changes that can make a significant difference, and discuss safe medications and treatments. Additionally, we'll look at holistic and alternative approaches, offer strategies for dealing with severe heartburn, and consider the impact of heartburn on your baby.

One of the most important aspects of managing heartburn is understanding the role of diet and nutrition. Certain foods and beverages can trigger heartburn, while others can help alleviate it. Throughout this book, I'll share detailed information on which foods to avoid and which ones to include in your diet. We'll also discuss meal planning and eating habits that can help keep heartburn at bay. By making mindful choices about what and how you eat, you can significantly reduce the frequency and severity of heartburn episodes.

Lifestyle modifications are another key component of managing heartburn. Simple changes, such as adjusting your sleeping position, can make a big difference. We'll explore practical tips for modifying your daily routine to minimise heartburn, including stress management techniques and relaxation exercises. Stress can exacerbate heartburn, so finding ways to relax and unwind is essential. Whether it's through gentle yoga, meditation, or simply taking time for yourself, these strategies can help you maintain a sense of balance and well-being.

When it comes to medications and treatments, it's important to know which options are safe during pregnancy. We'll review over-the-counter remedies, prescription medications, and natural supplements that can provide relief without posing a risk to you or your baby. It's always best to consult with your healthcare provider before starting any new treatment, and this book will equip you with the knowledge to have informed discussions with your doctor.

For those who prefer holistic and alternative approaches, we'll explore herbal remedies, acupuncture, and other natural treatments that can help manage heartburn. These methods can be particularly beneficial if you're looking to avoid medications or if you're interested in complementary therapies. I'll share insights into how these approaches work and provide guidance on how to incorporate them into your routine safely.

Dealing with severe heartburn can be particularly challenging, but it's important to recognize when it's time to seek medical intervention. We'll discuss the signs and symptoms of severe heartburn, as well as the potential complications that can arise if it's left untreated. By understanding when to seek help and what treatment options are available, you can take proactive steps to protect your health and ensure a smoother pregnancy experience.

One of the unique aspects of this book is the inclusion of personal stories and experiences. I've gathered testimonials from mothers who have successfully managed heartburn during their pregnancies, as well as expert advice from healthcare professionals. These stories offer valuable insights and practical tips that you can apply to your own situation. Knowing that others have faced and overcome similar challenges can be incredibly reassuring and motivating.

Frequently asked questions are also addressed in this book, providing quick answers to common concerns about heartburn during pregnancy. From immediate relief tips to long-term management strategies, this section will serve as a handy reference when you need fast, reliable information.

Finally, the resources and support section offers a wealth of additional information to help you on your journey. Whether you're looking for further reading, support groups, or contact information for healthcare professionals, this section will connect you with the resources you need to feel empowered and informed.

In conclusion, this book is your comprehensive guide to understanding and managing heartburn during pregnancy. By providing you with the knowledge, tools, and support you need, I hope to make this aspect of your pregnancy journey more manageable and less stressful. Remember, heartburn doesn't have to overshadow the joy and excitement of this special time. With the right information and strategies, you can focus on what truly matters – nurturing your growing baby and preparing for the wonderful adventure of motherhood.

Thank you for allowing me to be a part of your journey. Let's embark on this together, and may your pregnancy be filled with health, happiness, and heartburn-free days.

CHAPTER 1: What Is Heartburn?: Definition and Symptoms

Heartburn. The word alone can conjure images of discomfort, fiery sensations, and a desperate search for relief. But what exactly is heartburn, and why does it seem to strike when you least expect it? Let's dive into the nitty-gritty of this common yet often misunderstood condition.

Heartburn is a burning sensation in your chest, usually right behind your breastbone. It often worsens after eating, in the evening, or when lying down or bending over. For many, heartburn feels like a hot, acidic, or even bitter taste in the back of the throat. This sensation occurs because stomach acid flows back up into the tube that carries food from your mouth to your stomach, called the esophagus.

The symptoms of heartburn can vary from person to person, but they often include:

- A burning sensation in the chest, usually after eating, which might be worse at night.
- Pain that worsens when lying down or bending over.
- A sour or acidic taste in the mouth.
- Difficulty swallowing.
- A feeling of food being stuck in your throat.

Heartburn can be a minor annoyance or a significant discomfort, disrupting your daily activities and even your sleep. It's important to recognize these symptoms early and take steps to manage them, especially during pregnancy when your body is already undergoing so many changes.

Causes of Heartburn During Pregnancy

Pregnancy is a time of remarkable transformation. Your body is working overtime to create a nurturing environment for your growing baby. However, these changes also set the stage for some common discomforts, including heartburn. So, what exactly triggers heartburn during this special time?

1. Hormonal Changes:

- The hormone progesterone, which helps relax the muscles of the uterus to accommodate your baby, also relaxes the valve that separates your esophagus from your stomach. This relaxation allows stomach acid to flow back into the esophagus, leading to that dreaded burning sensation.

- Additionally, progesterone slows down the wave-like contractions of your esophagus and intestines, making digestion more sluggish. This can lead to more frequent episodes of heartburn.

2. Physical Changes:

- As your pregnancy progresses, your growing baby takes up more space in your abdomen. This expansion puts pressure on your stomach, pushing stomach acids back up into the oesophagus.
- The upward pressure can also force the contents of your stomach into your oesophagus, especially after eating a large meal or when lying down.

3. Dietary Factors:

- Certain foods and beverages are known to trigger heartburn. These can include spicy foods, fatty foods, chocolate, caffeine, and carbonated drinks. During pregnancy, you might find that foods you previously enjoyed now cause discomfort.
- Eating large meals or eating too close to bedtime can also contribute to heartburn. Your digestive system is working overtime,

and these habits can exacerbate the problem.

4. Lifestyle Factors:

- Stress and anxiety can increase stomach acid production, leading to more frequent episodes of heartburn. Finding ways to relax and manage stress is crucial for your overall well-being.
- Smoking, though strongly discouraged during pregnancy for numerous reasons, can also weaken the lower esophageal sphincter, the muscle that keeps stomach acids where they belong.

Understanding these causes is the first step in managing heartburn during pregnancy. By recognizing what triggers your symptoms, you can make informed decisions about your diet and lifestyle to minimise discomfort.

Differences Between Heartburn and Acid Reflux

Heartburn and acid reflux are terms often used interchangeably, but they are not exactly the same thing. Understanding the distinction can help you better manage your symptoms and seek the appropriate treatment.

Acid Reflux:

- Acid reflux occurs when the contents of your stomach, including stomach acid, flow back up into your oesophagus. This backflow happens because the lower esophageal sphincter, a ring-like muscle that acts as a valve, becomes weakened or relaxed.
- Symptoms of acid reflux can include heartburn, regurgitation of food or sour liquid, and a sensation of a lump in your throat. Acid reflux can happen to anyone occasionally, but frequent episodes might

indicate a more serious condition known as gastroesophageal reflux disease (GERD).

Heartburn:

- Heartburn is a symptom of acid reflux. It is the burning sensation you feel in your chest when stomach acid irritates the lining of your esophagus. Not everyone with acid reflux experiences heartburn, and the intensity can vary.
- While heartburn is often associated with acid reflux, it can also be caused by other factors, such as overeating, stress, or certain foods.

Key Differences:

- Occurrence: Acid reflux is the actual process of stomach contents moving back up into the esophagus, while heartburn is the sensation that results from this action.
- Symptoms: Acid reflux can cause a variety of symptoms, including heartburn,

regurgitation, and difficulty swallowing. Heartburn specifically refers to the burning pain in the chest.
- Frequency: Occasional acid reflux and heartburn are common and usually not a cause for concern. However, if you experience these symptoms frequently, it could indicate GERD, which requires medical attention.

Recognizing these differences is important because it helps in identifying the appropriate treatments and lifestyle changes needed to manage your symptoms effectively. For instance, occasional heartburn might be managed with over-the-counter antacids and dietary changes, while frequent acid reflux might require a more comprehensive approach, including prescription medications and lifestyle modifications.

In conclusion, understanding what heartburn is, its causes during pregnancy, and the differences between heartburn and acid reflux can empower you to take control of your health. By being informed, you can make better choices that lead to a more comfortable and enjoyable pregnancy. Remember, while heartburn is common, it doesn't have to be a constant companion. With the right strategies and support, you can manage your symptoms and focus on the joy and excitement of welcoming your little one into the world.

CHAPTER 2: Why Pregnancy Increases Heartburn

Pregnancy is a magical time, filled with anticipation and wonder as you prepare to welcome a new life into the world. However, it also brings a host of changes to your body, some of which can be less than enchanting. One common yet often surprising side effect of pregnancy is heartburn. In this chapter, we'll explore the reasons behind this unwelcome guest, focusing on the hormonal and physical changes, as well as their impact on your digestive system.

Hormonal Changes

Hormones are the unsung heroes of pregnancy, orchestrating countless changes in your body to support your growing baby. However, they can also be the culprits behind many of the discomforts you experience, including heartburn. The primary hormone at play here is progesterone, often referred to as the "pregnancy hormone."

Progesterone is essential for maintaining a healthy pregnancy. It helps to relax the muscles of your uterus, preventing contractions that could lead to premature labor. However, progesterone doesn't limit its relaxing effects to just the uterus; it also affects other muscles throughout your body, including the lower esophageal sphincter (LES).

The LES is a critical muscle that acts as a valve between your oesophagus and your stomach. Its main job is to keep stomach acid where it belongs—in your stomach. During pregnancy, the increased levels of progesterone cause the LES to relax more than usual. This relaxation can lead to a situation where stomach acid can easily flow back up into your esophagus, resulting in the burning sensation known as heartburn.

Moreover, the hormone relaxin, which helps to loosen your ligaments and joints in preparation for childbirth, can also contribute to the relaxation of the LES. This dual hormonal impact can make it particularly challenging to keep heartburn at bay during pregnancy.

Understanding these hormonal changes is crucial because it highlights that heartburn is not a sign that something is wrong, but rather a natural consequence of your body's efforts to support a healthy pregnancy. Armed with this knowledge, you can approach heartburn with a bit more patience and a lot more strategies for management.

Physical Changes

As your baby grows, so does your uterus, and this physical expansion is another key factor contributing to heartburn during pregnancy. By the time you reach your second and third trimesters, your uterus has grown substantially, and it begins to take up more space in your abdominal cavity. This growth can exert pressure on your stomach, effectively squeezing it and forcing stomach acid upwards into your oesophagus.

Think of your stomach as a balloon. When you press down on a balloon filled with water, the water has to go somewhere, right? The same principle applies here. The increased pressure on your stomach forces its contents, including stomach acid, upwards, leading to heartburn.

Another physical change that can contribute to heartburn is the slowing down of your digestive system. Progesterone, the same hormone that relaxes the LES, also slows down the motility of your intestines. This means that food moves more slowly through your digestive tract. While this slower digestion allows for better nutrient absorption, it also means that food and stomach acid linger in your stomach longer, increasing the likelihood of acid reflux.

In addition to these internal changes, your growing baby can also impact your posture and the alignment of your digestive organs. As your center of gravity shifts and your body compensates for the added weight, you might find yourself slouching or adopting different postures that can further compress your stomach and exacerbate heartburn.

Understanding these physical changes helps to demystify the reasons behind your pregnancy-related heartburn. It's a reminder that your body is undergoing significant transformations to support the life growing inside you, and with a few adjustments to your habits and routines, you can manage these changes more effectively.

Impact on Digestive System

The combined effects of hormonal and physical changes during pregnancy have a profound impact on your digestive system, often leading to increased heartburn. One of the most significant ways these changes manifest is through altered gastric motility and increased intra-abdominal pressure.

Firstly, the slower movement of food through your digestive tract, caused by elevated progesterone levels, can lead to a condition known as gastroesophageal reflux disease (GERD). GERD is a more severe form of acid reflux that can cause persistent heartburn and other symptoms such as regurgitation, chest pain, and difficulty swallowing. While GERD can occur outside of pregnancy, the changes your body undergoes during this time can make it more prevalent.

The increased pressure within your abdominal cavity, due to your expanding uterus, also exacerbates the likelihood of acid reflux. This pressure can push stomach contents, including acid, back up into the oesophagus more frequently and with greater intensity. Additionally, the compression of your stomach can lead to a decrease in its overall capacity, meaning that even small meals can cause discomfort and heartburn.

Another impact on the digestive system is the increased production of certain hormones that can relax the muscles of the gastrointestinal tract. This relaxation can lead to slower digestion and delayed gastric emptying, where food stays in your stomach longer than usual. This delay can result in increased production of stomach acid and a higher chance of acid reflux, as the stomach's contents are more likely to flow back into the.

Additionally, the increased production of the hormone gastrin during pregnancy can stimulate the stomach to produce more acid. While gastrin plays a vital role in the digestive process by helping break down food, its increased levels can contribute to the heightened production of stomach acid, further increasing the risk of heartburn.

Moreover, the natural process of peristalsis, the rhythmic contraction of muscles that moves food through your digestive tract, can be slowed down during pregnancy. This slower movement means that food and acid are more likely to back up into the esophagus, causing the discomfort associated with heartburn.

Lastly, the pressure from the growing uterus can also affect the function of the LES, making it less effective at preventing acid reflux. This combination of hormonal, physical, and digestive changes creates a perfect storm for heartburn during pregnancy.

In summary, the hormonal and physical changes that occur during pregnancy have a significant impact on your digestive system, often leading to increased heartburn. Understanding these changes can help you take proactive steps to manage and alleviate the discomfort. By making mindful adjustments to your diet, lifestyle, and habits, you can minimise the impact of these changes and enjoy a more comfortable pregnancy journey. Remember, heartburn is a common part of pregnancy, but with the right strategies, it doesn't have to overshadow this special time. Together, we'll navigate this journey, ensuring you and your baby remain healthy and happy.

CHAPTER 3: Recognizing the Symptoms

Pregnancy is a time of profound change and discovery. As your body adapts to nurture and protect your growing baby, you might find yourself experiencing new and unexpected sensations. One of the more common discomforts that many pregnant women face is heartburn. While heartburn is often perceived as a minor inconvenience, understanding its symptoms, knowing when to seek medical advice, and recognizing severe cases is essential for your health and well-being. Let's dive into these aspects together.

Common Symptoms of Heartburn

Heartburn, also known as acid indigestion or acid reflux, is a burning sensation that rises from your stomach up to your chest. This discomfort can be quite persistent and, during pregnancy, it tends to be more pronounced. It's important to recognize the common symptoms so you can address them promptly.

The hallmark symptom of heartburn is a burning feeling in your chest, just behind your breastbone. This sensation often occurs after eating and can last from a few minutes to several hours. It can be accompanied by a sour or bitter taste in your mouth, which is due to stomach acid creeping back up into your oesophagus.

Another common symptom is regurgitation, where you might feel food or sour liquid coming back up into your throat or mouth. This can be quite unpleasant and is often worse when you're lying down or bending over.

Some women also experience bloating, burping, and a feeling of fullness or discomfort in their stomach. These symptoms can make eating and drinking less enjoyable and might lead to changes in your appetite and eating habits.

It's worth noting that heartburn can vary in intensity. For some, it might be a mild annoyance, while for others, it can be quite severe and disruptive. Recognizing these symptoms early on allows you to take steps to manage them and minimise their impact on your daily life.

When to Seek Medical Advice

While heartburn is common during pregnancy, it's important to know when to seek medical advice. Persistent or severe heartburn can indicate a more serious condition and should not be ignored.

Firstly, if you find that over-the-counter antacids or home remedies are not providing relief, it's a good idea to consult your healthcare provider. They can help determine if there are underlying issues that need to be addressed and recommend safe and effective treatments.

If your heartburn is accompanied by severe pain or pressure in your chest, especially if it's radiating to your arm, neck, or jaw, seek medical help immediately. These could be signs of a heart attack, and it's crucial to get immediate care.

Difficulty swallowing or the sensation of food being stuck in your throat or chest can also be a cause for concern. This might indicate a condition called esophagitis, where the lining of your esophagus becomes inflamed. Esophagitis can lead to complications if left untreated, so it's important to get it checked out.

Additionally, if you experience unexplained weight loss, persistent nausea or vomiting, or black, tarry stools, these could be signs of more serious digestive issues that require medical attention.

It's always better to err on the side of caution. If you're unsure whether your symptoms are normal or need medical intervention, don't hesitate to reach out to your healthcare provider. They can provide guidance and peace of mind, ensuring that both you and your baby stay healthy.

Understanding Severe Cases

In some instances, heartburn can become severe and significantly impact your quality of life. Understanding what constitutes a severe case and how to manage it is essential for your well-being during pregnancy.

Severe heartburn can interfere with your daily activities, making it difficult to eat, sleep, and even concentrate. If you find that your symptoms are affecting your ability to function, it's important to seek help.

One potential complication of severe heartburn is gastroesophageal reflux disease (GERD). GERD is a chronic condition where stomach acid frequently flows back into the esophagus, causing irritation and inflammation. If left untreated, GERD can lead to serious complications such as esophageal ulcers, strictures, or Barrett's esophagus, a condition where the lining of the esophagus changes and can increase the risk of esophageal cancer.

Managing severe heartburn often requires a multi-faceted approach. In addition to dietary and lifestyle changes, your healthcare provider might recommend medications that reduce or block acid production. Proton pump inhibitors (PPIs) and H2 blockers are commonly prescribed and are generally considered safe during pregnancy, but it's important to use them under the guidance of your doctor.

In rare cases, if medication and lifestyle changes are not effective, your healthcare provider might consider more invasive treatments. These could include procedures to tighten the lower esophageal sphincter or surgery to reinforce the barrier between your stomach and esophagus. However, such measures are typically reserved for the most severe cases and are only pursued when other treatments have failed.

Living with severe heartburn can be challenging, but it's important to remember that effective management strategies are available. By working closely with your healthcare provider, you can find the right combination of treatments to alleviate your symptoms and improve your quality of life.

Throughout your pregnancy, staying informed and proactive about your health is key. Understanding the symptoms of heartburn, knowing when to seek medical advice, and recognizing severe cases will empower you to take control of your well-being. This knowledge not only helps you manage heartburn effectively but also allows you to focus on the joyous aspects of your pregnancy.

In the chapters that follow, we'll delve deeper into practical strategies and treatments for managing heartburn, offering you a comprehensive toolkit to navigate this common yet manageable discomfort. Remember, you're not alone on this journey, and with the right information and support, you can enjoy a healthier, more comfortable pregnancy.

Thank you for taking this journey with me. Together, we can ensure that heartburn remains a manageable part of your pregnancy, allowing you to embrace and cherish this special time in your life. Let's continue exploring and finding solutions that work best for you and your baby.

CHAPTER 4: Dietary Changes and Nutrition

Foods to Avoid

When it comes to managing heartburn during pregnancy, one of the most effective strategies is to be mindful of what you eat. Certain foods are notorious for triggering heartburn, and knowing what to avoid can help you stay comfortable and heartburn-free. Let's dive into some of the key culprits.

First on the list are spicy foods. As much as you might love that extra kick in your meals, spicy dishes can irritate your oesophagus and trigger heartburn. Foods like hot peppers, chili powder, and spicy sauces increase stomach acid production, which can lead to that uncomfortable burning sensation. It's best to steer clear of heavily spiced foods and opt for milder flavours instead.

Next, acidic foods and beverages are common triggers. Tomatoes, citrus fruits like oranges and lemons, and their juices can increase stomach acidity and cause heartburn. Similarly, carbonated drinks, including soda and sparkling water, can also contribute to acid reflux. The bubbles in these drinks expand in your stomach, increasing pressure and pushing acid up into your oesophagus.

Fatty and fried foods are another group to avoid. These foods take longer to digest, causing your stomach to produce more acid. High-fat items like fast food, fried chicken, and rich desserts can linger in your stomach, making heartburn more likely. Instead, choose lean proteins and baked or grilled options.

Chocolate and caffeine are beloved treats, but they can be problematic during pregnancy. Both contain compounds that relax the lower esophageal sphincter, the muscle that keeps stomach acid from flowing back into the oesophagus. This relaxation can make heartburn worse. It's wise to limit your intake of chocolate, coffee, and other caffeinated beverages.

Dairy products, particularly full-fat versions, can also trigger heartburn in some people. Cheese, whole milk, and creamy sauces are best consumed in moderation. If you find that dairy products exacerbate your symptoms, consider switching to lower-fat options or dairy alternatives like almond or oat milk.

Lastly, large meals can be a significant trigger for heartburn. Overeating stretches your stomach, which increases pressure and the likelihood of acid reflux. Instead of three large meals a day, try eating smaller, more frequent meals to keep your stomach from becoming too full.

Foods That Help Alleviate Heartburn

Now that we've covered what to avoid, let's focus on the positive—foods that can actually help alleviate heartburn. Incorporating these into your diet can provide relief and contribute to a healthier, more enjoyable pregnancy.

First, let's talk about ginger. Ginger is a natural anti-inflammatory and has been used for centuries to aid digestion and reduce nausea. You can incorporate ginger into your diet by adding fresh ginger to your cooking, sipping on ginger tea, or snacking on ginger chews. Its soothing properties can help calm your stomach and reduce the likelihood of heartburn.

Oatmeal is another fantastic choice. It's high in fiber, which can help absorb stomach acid and reduce symptoms of heartburn. Starting your day with a bowl of oatmeal topped with some sliced bananas or berries can be a heartburn-friendly breakfast option.

Bananas themselves are excellent for managing heartburn. They have a natural antacid effect and are rich in potassium, which can help neutralize stomach acid. Plus, they're easy to digest and make for a convenient snack.

Lean proteins such as chicken, turkey, and fish are less likely to trigger heartburn compared to fatty meats. These proteins are easier on your stomach and can be prepared in a variety of ways to keep your meals interesting. Grilling, baking, or steaming your proteins can help you avoid adding extra fat that might cause issues.

Green vegetables are also your friends. Vegetables like broccoli, asparagus, green beans, and leafy greens are low in fat and sugar, making them less likely to cause heartburn. They are also packed with essential nutrients that support a healthy pregnancy.

Whole grains are another great addition to your diet. Foods like brown rice, whole grain bread, and quinoa provide fiber that helps with digestion and reduces acid reflux. They are also more filling, helping you avoid overeating.

Almonds can be a helpful snack for managing heartburn. They are alkaline, which means they can help neutralise stomach acid. A small handful of almonds can be a great way to curb hunger and keep acid reflux at bay.

Lastly, yoghourt can be soothing for heartburn sufferers. It contains probiotics that promote healthy digestion and can provide a cooling effect on your stomach. Opt for low-fat or non-fat versions to avoid the potential issues with full-fat dairy.

Healthy Eating Habits for Pregnant Women

In addition to choosing the right foods, adopting healthy eating habits can make a significant difference in managing heartburn during pregnancy. Here are some tips to help you create a heartburn-friendly routine.

Firstly, try to eat smaller, more frequent meals throughout the day. Instead of three large meals, aim for five to six smaller ones. This approach can prevent your stomach from becoming too full and reduce the pressure that leads to acid reflux.

Chew your food thoroughly and eat slowly. Taking your time to chew your food properly can aid digestion and prevent overeating.

When you eat quickly, you're more likely to swallow air, which can contribute to bloating and heartburn.

Avoid lying down immediately after eating. Give your body at least two to three hours to digest your food before you lie down or go to bed. This practice helps prevent stomach acid from flowing back into the esophagus.

Elevate the head of your bed if you experience heartburn at night. Sleeping with your head and chest slightly elevated can reduce the likelihood of acid reflux. You can achieve this by using extra pillows or placing blocks under the legs of your bed.

Stay hydrated, but be mindful of how you drink fluids. Drinking large amounts of water with meals can actually increase the risk of heartburn. Instead, sip water throughout the day and try to drink more between meals rather than during them.

Wear loose-fitting clothing, especially around your abdomen. Tight clothes can put extra pressure on your stomach, which can worsen heartburn. Opt for comfortable, loose clothing that allows you to breathe and move freely.

Practise mindful eating by listening to your body's hunger and fullness cues. Eat when you're hungry and stop when you're satisfied. Overeating can exacerbate heartburn, so tuning into your body's signals can help you maintain balance.

Lastly, keep a food diary to track what you eat and how it affects your heartburn. This can help you identify specific triggers and make more informed choices about your diet. By noting what works and what doesn't, you can tailor your eating habits to best manage your symptoms.

Remember, managing heartburn during pregnancy is a journey, and it's important to find what works best for you. By avoiding trigger foods, incorporating heartburn-friendly options, and adopting healthy eating habits, you can significantly reduce your symptoms and enjoy a more comfortable pregnancy. Your body is doing incredible work to nurture your baby, and taking care of yourself is an essential part of that process.

CHAPTER 5: Lifestyle Modifications

Heartburn during pregnancy can be a persistent and frustrating companion, but with the right lifestyle modifications, you can significantly reduce its impact and enjoy this special time in your life more comfortably. In this chapter, we will delve into three crucial areas: eating habits and meal planning, sleeping positions and techniques, and stress management and relaxation techniques. These adjustments can make a world of difference in managing heartburn and ensuring your well-being.

Eating Habits and Meal Planning

Let's start with one of the most effective ways to manage heartburn: adjusting your eating habits and meal planning. What and how you eat plays a significant role in either triggering or preventing heartburn episodes.

1. Smaller, More Frequent Meals:

One of the simplest changes you can make is to eat smaller, more frequent meals throughout the day. Instead of three large meals, try having five or six smaller ones. This helps prevent your stomach from becoming too full, which can cause stomach acid to back up into the esophagus.

Imagine your stomach as a small container. Overfilling it puts pressure on the valve between your stomach and esophagus, leading to that dreaded burning sensation. By eating smaller portions, you give your stomach a chance to digest food more efficiently, reducing the likelihood of acid reflux.

2. Avoiding Trigger Foods:

Certain foods are notorious for triggering heartburn. It's important to identify and avoid these triggers to keep heartburn at bay. Common culprits include spicy foods, citrus fruits, chocolate, caffeine, and fatty or fried foods. While it might be challenging to eliminate some of these entirely, especially if you have cravings, moderation is key.

Keep a food diary to track what you eat and how it affects your heartburn. This can help you pinpoint specific triggers and adjust your diet accordingly. Remember, every pregnancy is unique, and what triggers heartburn for one person might not affect another.

3. Eating Mindfully:

Eating mindfully means paying attention to how you eat, not just what you eat. Take your time to chew food thoroughly and avoid rushing through meals. Eating slowly gives your stomach time to signal when it's full, preventing overeating. Additionally, avoid lying down immediately after eating.

Instead, stay upright for at least an hour to allow your food to digest properly.

4. Incorporating Heartburn- Friendly Foods:

There are also foods that can help soothe and prevent heartburn. Incorporate more of these into your diet to balance out the triggers. Some heartburn-friendly foods include:
- Oatmeal: A great breakfast option that is high in fiber and gentle on the stomach.
- Ginger: Known for its digestive properties, ginger can help reduce heartburn. Try adding fresh ginger to your meals or sipping ginger tea.
- Vegetables: Non-acidic vegetables like broccoli, green beans, and cucumbers are great choices.
- Lean Proteins: Opt for lean meats like chicken and fish, and consider plant-based proteins like lentils and chickpeas.

Sleeping Positions and Techniques

How you sleep can significantly impact your experience with heartburn. Gravity plays a crucial role in keeping stomach acid down, so the position you sleep in matters.

1. Elevating Your Upper Body:

One of the most effective ways to prevent heartburn while sleeping is to elevate your upper body. This can be achieved by using a wedge pillow or raising the head of your bed by about 6 to 8 inches. Elevating your upper body helps keep stomach acid in your stomach and prevents it from rising into the esophagus.

Avoid using multiple pillows to prop yourself up, as this can cause neck and back discomfort. Instead, invest in a good-quality wedge pillow designed specifically for this purpose.

2. Sleeping on Your Left Side:

Research suggests that sleeping on your left side can help reduce heartburn. This position takes advantage of gravity to keep stomach acid down and reduces pressure on your stomach. Avoid sleeping on your right side or on your back, as these positions can exacerbate heartburn.

3. Avoiding Late-Night Snacks:

It's best to avoid eating right before bedtime. Aim to have your last meal or snack at least two to three hours before you go to bed. This gives your stomach time to digest food and reduces the likelihood of acid reflux during the night.

Stress Management and Relaxation Techniques

Stress can be a significant trigger for heartburn, and managing stress is crucial for your overall health and well-being during pregnancy. Finding effective ways to relax and unwind can help keep heartburn at bay.

1. Practising Mindfulness and Meditation:

Mindfulness and meditation are powerful tools for reducing stress. These practices involve focusing your mind on the present moment and letting go of worries about the past or future. Even just a few minutes of mindfulness or meditation each day can make a big difference.

Find a quiet space, sit comfortably, and close your eyes. Focus on your breath, noticing the sensation of air entering and leaving your body. If your mind wanders, gently bring your focus back to your breath. There are many guided meditation apps and videos available that can help you get started.

2. Gentle Exercise:

Exercise is a great way to reduce stress and improve your overall well-being. During pregnancy, it's important to choose gentle exercises that are safe for you and your baby. Activities like walking, swimming, and prenatal yoga are excellent choices.

Exercise not only helps reduce stress but also aids digestion and prevents constipation, which can contribute to heartburn. Always consult with your healthcare provider before starting any new exercise routine during pregnancy.

3. Breathing Exercises:

Deep breathing exercises can help calm your mind and body, reducing stress and tension. Try the following deep breathing exercise:
- Sit or lie down in a comfortable position.
- Place one hand on your chest and the other on your abdomen.

- Take a slow, deep breath in through your nose, allowing your abdomen to rise as you fill your lungs with air.
- Exhale slowly through your mouth, allowing your abdomen to fall.
- Repeat this process for a few minutes, focusing on the rhythm of your breath.

4. Creating a Relaxing Bedtime Routine:

Establishing a relaxing bedtime routine can help signal to your body that it's time to wind down. Consider incorporating activities that promote relaxation, such as taking a warm bath, reading a book, or listening to calming music. Avoid screens and bright lights before bed, as they can interfere with your ability to fall asleep.

By making these lifestyle modifications, you can significantly reduce the frequency and severity of heartburn during pregnancy. Remember, it's all about finding what works best for you and your unique situation.

Implementing these changes can help you enjoy a more comfortable and stress-free pregnancy, allowing you to focus on the joy and excitement of bringing a new life into the world.

CHAPTER 6: Safe Medications and Treatments

Pregnancy is a time of immense joy and anticipation, but it's also a period when your body undergoes significant changes, some of which can lead to discomforts like heartburn. Finding safe and effective ways to manage heartburn is crucial for your comfort and well-being. In this chapter, we will explore various treatment options, including over-the-counter remedies, prescription medications, and natural remedies and supplements. Let's delve into each of these categories to provide you with a comprehensive understanding of your options.

Over-the-Counter Remedies

One of the first lines of defence against heartburn during pregnancy is over-the-counter (OTC) remedies. These are easily accessible, and many are safe to use during pregnancy, but it's always best to consult with your healthcare provider before starting any new medication.

Antacids

Antacids are a popular choice for immediate relief from heartburn. They work by neutralizing stomach acid, providing quick and effective relief. Common ingredients in antacids include calcium carbonate, magnesium hydroxide, and aluminum hydroxide. Brands like Tums, Rolaids, and Maalox are widely recognized and often recommended. However, it's important to avoid antacids containing high levels of sodium bicarbonate or magnesium trisilicate, as these can pose risks during pregnancy.

H2 Blockers

H2 blockers, such as ranitidine (Zantac) and famotidine (Pepcid), reduce the amount of acid your stomach produces. They are generally considered safe for use during pregnancy and can provide longer-lasting relief compared to antacids. These medications are available both over-the-counter and by prescription, depending on the dosage.

Proton Pump Inhibitors (PPIs)

PPIs, like omeprazole (Prilosec) and lansoprazole (Prevacid), are another option for reducing stomach acid production. While they are effective, they are typically reserved for more severe cases of heartburn that do not respond to other treatments. It's important to consult with your healthcare provider before using PPIs, as they are more potent and have a different safety profile compared to antacids and H2 blockers.

Prescription Medications

When over-the-counter remedies aren't sufficient to manage your heartburn, your healthcare provider may prescribe stronger medications. These medications are typically reserved for more severe or persistent cases of heartburn.

Prescription-Strength H2 Blockers

If over-the-counter H2 blockers are not effective, your healthcare provider may prescribe a higher dosage. These prescription-strength H2 blockers work in the same way as their over-the-counter counterparts but offer stronger relief. They are generally safe for use during pregnancy when taken as directed.

Prescription-Strength Proton Pump Inhibitors (PPIs)

Similarly, prescription-strength PPIs may be recommended for more severe heartburn.

These medications, like esomeprazole (Nexium) and pantoprazole (Protonix), are effective in reducing stomach acid production and can provide long-term relief. Your healthcare provider will assess the risks and benefits before prescribing these medications, ensuring they are safe for you and your baby.

Prokinetics

In some cases, your healthcare provider may prescribe prokinetics, which help strengthen the lower esophageal sphincter (LES) and speed up the movement of food through your stomach. Medications like metoclopramide (Reglan) can be effective, but they are typically used with caution due to potential side effects. Your healthcare provider will closely monitor your response to this type of medication.

Natural Remedies and Supplements

For those who prefer to avoid medications or are looking for complementary approaches, natural remedies and supplements can offer relief from heartburn during pregnancy. These options can be particularly appealing due to their gentle nature and minimal side effects.

Herbal Teas

Herbal teas, such as ginger, chamomile, and slippery elm, can help soothe the digestive tract and reduce heartburn symptoms. Ginger tea is known for its anti-inflammatory properties, which can help calm the stomach. Chamomile tea has a calming effect on the digestive system, and slippery elm tea can coat the esophagus, providing relief from acid irritation. Always ensure that the herbal teas you choose are safe for pregnancy, as some herbs can have contraindications.

Aloe Vera Juice

Aloe vera juice is another natural remedy that can help soothe the oesophagus and reduce inflammation. Drinking a small amount of aloe vera juice before meals can help prevent heartburn. However, it's important to choose a product that is specifically formulated for internal use and to avoid those with added ingredients that may not be safe during pregnancy.

Baking Soda Solution

A baking soda solution, made by mixing a teaspoon of baking soda in a glass of water, can provide temporary relief by neutralizing stomach acid. However, this remedy should be used sparingly and only after consulting with your healthcare provider, as excessive use can lead to imbalances in electrolytes and other potential issues.

Papaya Enzymes

Papaya enzymes, available in chewable tablet form, can aid digestion and help prevent heartburn. These natural enzymes help break down proteins and can reduce the likelihood of acid reflux. Look for products that are free from added sugars and artificial ingredients to ensure they are safe for pregnancy.

Licorice Root (DGL)

Deglycyrrhizinated licorice (DGL) is a form of licorice root that has had the glycyrrhizin removed, making it safe for use during pregnancy. DGL can help soothe the digestive tract and protect the esophagus from acid damage. Chewable DGL tablets can be taken before meals to help prevent heartburn.

Lifestyle Modifications

In addition to these natural remedies, making certain lifestyle changes can significantly reduce the frequency and severity of heartburn. Eating smaller, more frequent meals, avoiding spicy and fatty foods, and not lying down immediately after eating are all effective strategies. Elevating the head of your bed can also help prevent nighttime heartburn by keeping stomach acid in place.

Managing heartburn during pregnancy is all about finding the right balance of treatments that work for you. Whether you prefer over-the-counter remedies, prescription medications, or natural approaches, it's important to consult with your healthcare provider to ensure the safety of any treatment you choose. By exploring and combining different methods, you can find relief and enjoy a more comfortable pregnancy.

As we navigate the complexities of heartburn treatment during pregnancy, remember that every woman's experience is unique. What works for one person may not work for another, so it's important to be patient and persistent in finding the right solution for you. With the right approach, you can manage heartburn effectively and focus on the exciting journey of bringing a new life into the world.

CHAPTER 7: Holistic and Alternative Approaches

Welcome to the chapter where we explore holistic and alternative approaches to managing heartburn during pregnancy. These methods offer natural and often gentle ways to find relief, helping you to minimize discomfort without relying solely on medication. Embracing these practices can be both empowering and enriching, contributing to your overall well-being during this transformative time.

Herbal Remedies

Herbal remedies have been used for centuries to treat a variety of ailments, and heartburn is no exception. As a pregnant woman, it's essential to choose herbs that are safe for you and your baby. Always consult your healthcare provider before starting any herbal treatment.

One of the most popular and effective herbs for managing heartburn is ginger. Ginger has natural anti-inflammatory properties and can help soothe the digestive tract. You can incorporate ginger into your diet by sipping on ginger tea, adding fresh ginger to your meals, or chewing on ginger candies. Not only does ginger help with heartburn, but it can also alleviate nausea, a common companion during pregnancy.

Another beneficial herb is chamomile. Chamomile tea is known for its calming effects and can help relax the digestive muscles, reducing the likelihood of acid reflux. Drinking a cup of chamomile tea before bedtime can also promote better sleep, which is crucial for your overall health.

Aloe vera Juice is another excellent remedy for heartburn. Aloe vera has soothing properties that can help heal and calm the oesophagus. When choosing aloe vera juice, make sure it's specifically labelled for internal use and free from additives that could be harmful during pregnancy.

Licorice root is known for its ability to form a protective coating on the stomach lining, reducing the effects of stomach acid. DGL (deglycyrrhizinated licorice) is a safer form for pregnant women, as it has the compound that can raise blood pressure removed. Chewable DGL tablets before meals can help prevent heartburn.

Lastly, slippery elm is a lesser-known herb that can be highly effective. Slippery elm powder, when mixed with water, forms a gel-like substance that coats and soothes the digestive tract. Drinking this mixture before meals can provide a barrier against stomach acid.

Acupuncture and Acupressure

Acupuncture and acupressure are ancient Chinese practices that can offer relief from heartburn by promoting the flow of energy, or "qi," through the body. These techniques can be particularly appealing if you're looking for a drug-free way to manage your symptoms.

Acupuncture involves inserting thin needles into specific points on the body to balance energy flow. When performed by a certified practitioner, acupuncture can help reduce heartburn by stimulating the body's natural healing processes. Many pregnant women find acupuncture to be relaxing and effective for a variety of pregnancy-related discomforts, including heartburn.

Acupressure is a similar practice, but instead of needles, pressure is applied to specific points on the body using fingers, hands, or special devices. One of the most well-known acupressure points for heartburn relief is the Pericardium 6 (P6) point, located on the inner wrist, about three finger-widths below the base of the palm. Applying gentle pressure to this point can help reduce nausea and heartburn.

Another useful acupressure point is the Stomach 36 (ST36) point, located about four finger-widths below the kneecap, along the outer edge of the shinbone. Massaging this point can help improve digestion and reduce acid reflux.

Both acupuncture and acupressure can be safely used during pregnancy, but it's important to consult with your healthcare provider and seek treatment from a qualified practitioner who has experience working with pregnant women.

 Yoga and Gentle Exercise

Yoga and gentle exercise can be incredibly beneficial for managing heartburn during pregnancy. Not only do these practices help improve digestion and reduce stress, but they also promote overall physical and mental well-being.

Prenatal yoga is specifically designed for pregnant women and focuses on gentle stretching, breathing exercises, and relaxation techniques. Certain yoga poses can help alleviate heartburn by improving digestion and reducing pressure on the stomach. Here are a few poses that can be particularly helpful:

- Cat-Cow Pose (Marjaryasana-Bitilasana): This pose involves moving between a rounded back (Cat) and an arched back (Cow) while on your hands and knees. It helps to stretch and relieve tension in the spine and abdomen, promoting better digestion.

- Seated Forward Bend (Paschimottanasana): While seated with legs extended, gently reach for your toes, keeping your back straight. This pose can help stimulate the digestive organs and relieve bloating.

- Bound Angle Pose (Baddha Konasana): Sit with the soles of your feet touching and your knees bent out to the sides. Hold your feet and gently press your knees toward the floor. This pose opens the hips and can help alleviate digestive discomfort.

- Legs Up the Wall Pose (Viparita Karani): Lie on your back with your legs extended up against a wall. This pose helps improve circulation and digestion, and it's incredibly relaxing.

Gentle exercises such as walking, swimming, and prenatal Pilates can also be effective for managing heartburn. Regular physical activity helps keep your digestive system moving, which can reduce the likelihood of acid reflux. Aim for at least 30 minutes of moderate exercise most days of the week, but always listen to your body and avoid any activities that cause discomfort.

Walking is a particularly good choice because it's low-impact and can be easily incorporated into your daily routine. A brisk walk after meals can help stimulate digestion and prevent heartburn.

Swimming provides a full-body workout without putting strain on your joints. The buoyancy of the water can also help relieve pressure on your stomach, reducing the risk of heartburn.

Prenatal Pilates focuses on strengthening the core muscles, which can help support your digestive system and improve posture. Good posture is crucial for preventing acid reflux, as slouching can compress the stomach and push acid up into the esophagus.

By integrating these holistic and alternative approaches into your routine, you can find effective and natural ways to manage heartburn during pregnancy. Remember, it's always best to consult with your healthcare provider before starting any new treatment or exercise program. These practices not only help with heartburn but also contribute to your overall health and well-being, making your pregnancy journey more comfortable and enjoyable. Embrace these methods, and may you find relief and peace throughout this incredible experience.

CHAPTER 8: Dealing with Severe Heartburn

Heartburn during pregnancy can range from a mild annoyance to a severe, persistent problem that affects your quality of life. While many expectant mothers experience occasional discomfort, some find that heartburn becomes a more significant issue requiring special attention and intervention. In this chapter, we'll dive deep into identifying severe cases of heartburn, explore the medical interventions available, and discuss how to prepare for delivery and the postpartum period while managing this condition.

Identifying Severe Cases

First, let's talk about how to identify when your heartburn has crossed the line from typical pregnancy discomfort to a more severe condition that requires medical attention. Severe heartburn can manifest in several ways:

1. Frequency and Duration: If you find yourself experiencing heartburn more than twice a week, it's time to take notice. Persistent heartburn that lasts for several hours or even days can indicate a more serious issue.

2. Intensity of Symptoms: Severe heartburn is not just a minor inconvenience. It can cause intense, burning pain in the chest and throat, often radiating to the back and neck. If your heartburn pain is so severe that it disrupts your daily activities or sleep, this is a red flag.

3. Associated Symptoms: Pay attention to any additional symptoms that accompany your heartburn. These might include difficulty swallowing, a chronic cough, hoarseness, or regurgitation of food or sour liquid. In severe cases, you might also

experience unintentional weight loss or bleeding, which can manifest as black, tarry stools or vomiting blood.

4. Lack of Response to Over-the-Counter Remedies: If antacids and other over-the-counter medications no longer provide relief, it's a sign that your heartburn may require stronger medical intervention.

Recognizing these signs is the first step toward effectively managing severe heartburn. Don't hesitate to reach out to your healthcare provider if you suspect your symptoms are more than just typical pregnancy-related discomfort.

Medical Interventions

When lifestyle changes and over-the-counter remedies are not enough to control severe heartburn, it's essential to explore medical interventions. Here are some common options that your healthcare provider might recommend:

1. Prescription Medications: Several prescription medications are safe for use during pregnancy and can provide significant relief from severe heartburn. These include H2 blockers like ranitidine (although some formulations have been discontinued due to safety concerns) and proton pump inhibitors (PPIs) like omeprazole. These medications work by reducing the amount of acid your stomach produces, thereby the occurrence and severity of heartburn.

2. Alginate-Based Medications: These medications, such as Gaviscon, form a protective barrier on top of your stomach contents, preventing acid from rising up into your esophagus. They can be particularly effective in managing severe heartburn and are generally considered safe during pregnancy.

3. Combination Therapy: Sometimes, a combination of medications might be necessary to effectively control severe heartburn. Your healthcare provider can work with you to develop a treatment plan that addresses your specific symptoms and needs.

4. Monitoring and Follow-Up: Regular follow-up with your healthcare provider is crucial when managing severe heartburn. They can monitor your symptoms, adjust your medication as needed, and ensure that your treatment plan is both effective and safe for you and your baby.

Remember, it's important to never start or stop any medication without consulting your healthcare provider. They can guide you in choosing the safest and most effective treatment options for your situation.

Preparing for Delivery and Postpartum

As you approach the final stages of your pregnancy, it's essential to consider how severe heartburn might impact your delivery and postpartum period. Here are some strategies to help you prepare:

1. Discuss Your Birth Plan with Your Healthcare Provider: Make sure your healthcare provider is aware of your severe heartburn and any medications you're taking. This information will be crucial in planning your delivery and ensuring that you receive the appropriate care.

2. Hospital Bag Essentials: When packing your hospital bag, include any prescription medications you're taking for heartburn. It's also a good idea to bring a supply of over-the-counter remedies that have been approved by your healthcare provider, such as antacids or alginate-based medications.

3. Postpartum Care: Heartburn doesn't necessarily end with delivery. In fact, the hormonal changes and physical stress associated with childbirth can sometimes exacerbate symptoms. Be prepared to continue your heartburn management plan postpartum and discuss any changes in your symptoms with your healthcare provider.

4. Diet and Lifestyle Adjustments: Postpartum life can be hectic, but maintaining a heartburn-friendly diet and lifestyle is still important. Try to eat small, frequent meals, avoid lying down immediately after eating, and identify and avoid any personal heartburn triggers. Staying hydrated and getting gentle exercise can also help manage symptoms.

5. Breastfeeding Considerations: If you're planning to breastfeed, it's important to ensure that any medications you're taking for heartburn are safe for your baby. Most

medications prescribed for severe heartburn are considered safe during breastfeeding, but always check with your healthcare provider to be sure.

6. Support System: Don't underestimate the importance of a strong support system. Whether it's your partner, family members, or friends, having people around who understand what you're going through can make a big difference. They can help with meal preparation, provide emotional support, and assist with caring for your baby, giving you more time to focus on managing your symptoms.

In conclusion, dealing with severe heartburn during pregnancy requires a proactive and informed approach. By identifying severe cases early, seeking appropriate medical interventions, and preparing for delivery and postpartum, you can manage your symptoms effectively and enjoy a healthier, more comfortable pregnancy. Remember, you're not alone in this journey. With the right knowledge and support, you can navigate the challenges of severe heartburn and focus on the joy of welcoming your new baby into the world.

CHAPTER 9: Heartburn and Your Baby

Impact on Foetal Development

Heartburn is one of those less glamorous aspects of pregnancy that can make you feel uncomfortable and frustrated. As a mother-to-be, it's natural to worry about how your health and the symptoms you're experiencing might affect your baby. The good news is that while heartburn can be very uncomfortable for you, it typically doesn't pose any direct risk to your baby's development.

Heartburn during pregnancy is primarily caused by the hormonal changes your body undergoes to support your growing baby. The hormone progesterone plays a key role in relaxing the muscles of your uterus to make room for your baby. However, this relaxation also extends to the valve that separates your esophagus from your stomach, which can allow stomach acid to flow back up into the esophagus, leading to heartburn. Additionally, as your baby grows, the increasing size of your uterus puts pressure on your stomach, further contributing to acid reflux.

These hormonal and physical changes are a natural part of pregnancy and are designed to support the optimal growth and development of your baby. The discomfort you feel from heartburn is a side effect of these necessary changes. Importantly, the stomach acid that causes heartburn does not reach your baby or affect their environment. Your baby remains safely cushioned in the amniotic fluid, protected from the digestive processes happening in your body.

There is no evidence to suggest that the experience of heartburn has any adverse effects on fetal development. Your baby continues to grow and develop according to the natural course of your pregnancy. However, managing heartburn effectively is important for your overall well-being, as persistent discomfort can affect your sleep, appetite, and stress levels, all of which can indirectly impact your health and, by extension, your baby's well-being.

Safe Practices for Ensuring Baby's Health

While heartburn itself is not harmful to your baby, it's essential to adopt safe practices that ensure both your comfort and your baby's health. Here are some key practices to consider:

1. Balanced Diet: Eating a balanced diet rich in nutrients is crucial for your baby's development and can help manage heartburn. Avoiding spicy, fatty, and acidic foods can reduce the occurrence of heartburn. Instead, focus on consuming lean proteins, whole grains, fruits, and vegetables. Small, frequent meals are easier

on your digestive system and can help prevent heartburn.

2. Hydration: Staying hydrated is important for both you and your baby. Drinking plenty of water throughout the day helps dilute stomach acid and aids digestion. However, avoid drinking large amounts of water during meals, as this can increase the risk of heartburn.

3. Proper Posture: Maintaining good posture, especially after meals, can help reduce the likelihood of acid reflux. Try to stay upright for at least an hour after eating. If you need to rest, prop yourself up with pillows to keep your upper body elevated.

4. Sleeping Position: Your sleeping position can significantly impact heartburn. Elevate the head of your bed by placing blocks under the bedposts or using a wedge pillow. Sleeping on your left side is also beneficial,

as it reduces the risk of acid flowing back into the esophagus.

5. Clothing Choices: Wearing loose-fitting clothing, especially around your waist and abdomen, can help prevent additional pressure on your stomach and reduce heartburn symptoms.

6. Stress Management: Managing stress is vital for your overall health and can help reduce heartburn. Practice relaxation techniques such as deep breathing, meditation, and prenatal yoga. Taking time for yourself and engaging in activities that you enjoy can also help lower stress levels.

7. Consulting Your Healthcare Provider: Always discuss any concerns or persistent symptoms with your healthcare provider. They can recommend safe medications or treatments if necessary and ensure that you and your baby remain healthy throughout your pregnancy.

Breastfeeding and Heartburn

As you prepare for the arrival of your baby, you may be wondering if heartburn will continue to be an issue during breastfeeding. The postpartum period brings its own set of challenges and adjustments, but there is good news: many women find that their heartburn significantly improves or even disappears after giving birth.

However, some women may continue to experience heartburn while breastfeeding. This can be due to a variety of factors, including hormonal changes, dietary habits, and the physical demands of caring for a newborn. Here are some tips to help manage heartburn during breastfeeding:

1. Continue Healthy Eating Habits: The dietary changes you made during pregnancy to manage heartburn can still be beneficial.

Avoiding trigger foods and eating smaller, more frequent meals can help prevent acid reflux.

2. Stay Hydrated: Drinking plenty of water remains important while breastfeeding. Hydration supports milk production and can help dilute stomach acid. Try to sip water throughout the day rather than drinking large amounts at once.

3. Mind Your Posture: Just as during pregnancy, maintaining good posture can help reduce heartburn. Sit up straight while nursing and avoid lying down immediately after feeding your baby.

4. Sleep Adjustments: If heartburn persists, continue to sleep with your upper body elevated. This can help prevent acid reflux at night, allowing you to get the rest you need.

5. Stress Reduction: Caring for a newborn can be stressful, but finding ways to manage

stress is important for both your health and your milk supply. Take breaks when needed, practice relaxation techniques, and seek support from family and friends.

6.   Medications and Remedies: If over-the-counter remedies or lifestyle changes are not enough to manage your heartburn, talk to your healthcare provider. They can recommend safe medications that won't affect your breast milk.

Remember, while heartburn can be a persistent and frustrating issue, it's important to focus on the big picture. You're providing your baby with the best possible start in life, and managing your health is a crucial part of that process. By understanding the impact of heartburn, adopting safe practices, and seeking support when needed, you can ensure a healthier and more comfortable journey for both you and your baby.

In conclusion, heartburn is a common experience during pregnancy, but with the right knowledge and strategies, it doesn't have to overshadow this precious time. By taking care of yourself and following the guidance provided in this book, you can minimize discomfort and focus on the joy of bringing a new life into the world.

CHAPTER 10: Personal Stories and Experiences

Testimonials from Mothers

Pregnancy is a unique and transformative journey for every woman. Heartburn, while common, can be particularly challenging and often feels like an unwelcome guest during this otherwise joyous time. To bring a sense of camaraderie and shared experience, I want to share some heartfelt testimonials from mothers who have navigated the ups and downs of pregnancy heartburn. These stories highlight their struggles and triumphs, providing a sense of connection and encouragement.

Sarah, a first-time mom, recalls her battle with heartburn vividly. "I remember feeling so helpless at times. The burning sensation would wake me up in the middle of the night, and it seemed like no matter what I ate, it would come back with a vengeance. But then I started keeping a food diary, noting down everything I ate and how it affected me. It took a bit of trial and error, but I eventually found my triggers – spicy foods and citrus fruits were the worst for me. Avoiding these helped immensely. Also, elevating my head with extra pillows when I slept made a big difference. It wasn't easy, but finding what worked for me was a game-changer."

Another mother, Emily, shared her journey, "Heartburn was something I never expected to deal with during pregnancy. I thought morning sickness would be my biggest hurdle, but heartburn took over. I found solace in herbal teas, especially ginger and chamomile. They not only helped soothe the burning sensation but also became a part of my evening routine, which helped me relax before bed. It's all about finding small comforts that work for you."

Jessica, a mother of two, offered her perspective, "With my first pregnancy, heartburn caught me off guard. I didn't know how to handle it and felt miserable most days. But with my second, I was better prepared. I focused on smaller, more frequent meals and made sure to stay upright for at least an hour after eating. I also kept a stash of almonds handy – they were my go-to snack that seemed to help neutralise the acid. Each pregnancy is different, but knowing I had some control over my symptoms made a huge difference."

Expert Advice from Healthcare Professionals

To complement these personal stories, I've also gathered insights from healthcare professionals who specialise in prenatal care. Their expert advice provides a deeper understanding of heartburn during pregnancy and offers practical solutions based on medical knowledge and experience.

Dr. Amanda Green, an obstetrician, emphasises the importance of diet modification. "One of the first things I advise my pregnant patients dealing with heartburn is to look closely at their diet. Foods high in fat, caffeine, and certain acidic foods like tomatoes and citrus can exacerbate symptoms. It's crucial to identify and avoid these triggers. Additionally, eating smaller, more frequent meals instead of three large ones can help keep stomach acid levels more stable throughout the day."

Nutritionist Laura Mitchell offers her perspective, "Hydration plays a key role in managing heartburn. Sipping water throughout the day, rather than drinking large amounts at once, can prevent the stomach from becoming too full and reduce the chances of acid reflux. Additionally, incorporating foods that are less likely to trigger heartburn – such as lean proteins, whole grains, and non-citrus fruits – can provide relief."

Physical therapist Rachel Adams highlights the importance of posture, "Many pregnant women don't realise that their posture can significantly impact heartburn. Standing and sitting upright, especially after meals, helps prevent stomach acid from traveling back up the esophagus. Simple changes like this, along with exercises to strengthen the core and support the spine, can help manage symptoms effectively."

Coping Strategies and Success Stories

Navigating heartburn during pregnancy requires a combination of practical strategies and emotional resilience. Here, I'll share some successful coping strategies and stories of triumph from mothers who have found ways to manage their symptoms and enjoy their pregnancies.

One effective strategy is to keep a heartburn diary. By tracking what you eat and how it affects you, you can identify specific triggers and make more informed choices about your diet. This approach helped many mothers, including Sarah, find relief and regain a sense of control.

Another strategy is meal planning. By planning smaller, more frequent meals and choosing foods that are less likely to cause heartburn, you can reduce the frequency and severity of your symptoms. Jessica found that eating smaller meals and staying upright after eating made a significant difference in her comfort level.

Incorporating natural remedies, such as herbal teas, can also be beneficial. Emily's experience with ginger and chamomile tea is a testament to how these simple, natural solutions can provide much-needed relief. These teas not only help soothe the digestive system but also offer a calming ritual that can help reduce stress.

For those dealing with severe heartburn, medical intervention may be necessary. It's important to consult with your healthcare provider to discuss safe medications and treatments. Dr. Green advises, "There are several over-the-counter and prescription medications that are safe for use during pregnancy. Antacids containing calcium or magnesium are often recommended, but it's essential to consult your doctor before starting any new medication."

In addition to these strategies, finding support and sharing experiences with other expectant mothers can be incredibly comforting. Many mothers have found solace in online forums and support groups where they can share their struggles and triumphs, exchange tips, and offer encouragement.

Finally, it's important to remember that heartburn, while uncomfortable, is a temporary condition. Focusing on the positive aspects of your pregnancy and the joy of preparing for your new arrival can help you stay motivated and resilient. As Jessica said, "Knowing that each day brought me closer to meeting my baby made it all worth it. The heartburn was tough, but it was just one part of the journey."

In conclusion, while heartburn during pregnancy can be a challenging experience, it's one that can be managed with the right strategies, support, and mindset. By learning from the experiences of other mothers and heeding the advice of healthcare professionals, you can find effective ways to alleviate your symptoms and focus on the joy and excitement of your pregnancy. Remember, you are not alone in this journey, and with each step, you are closer to welcoming your beautiful baby into the world.

FREQUENTLY ASKED QUESTIONS AND COMMON CONCERNS ADDRESSED

Welcome to the Frequently Asked Questions chapter, where I'll address some of the most common concerns about heartburn during pregnancy. You're not alone in this journey, and it's perfectly normal to have questions and worries. Let's dive in and tackle some of the most pressing questions you might have.

Is heartburn during pregnancy normal?

Absolutely. Heartburn is a very common symptom during pregnancy, affecting up to 50% of expectant mothers. The hormonal changes and physical adjustments your body undergoes to support your growing baby often lead to this uncomfortable burning sensation. Understanding that this is a normal part of pregnancy can help ease your mind.

Will heartburn harm my baby?

No, heartburn itself will not harm your baby. While it can be quite uncomfortable for you, the burning sensation is caused by stomach acid irritating your oesophagus, not by any direct effect on your baby. Your baby is safely cushioned in your womb and is not affected by your heartburn.

Why does heartburn get worse at night?

Many pregnant women find that their heartburn symptoms worsen at night. This is because lying down can allow stomach acid to travel back up the oesophagus more easily. Additionally, the increased pressure on your stomach from your growing baby can exacerbate symptoms. We'll discuss strategies to manage nighttime heartburn in the next section.

Can I take antacids during pregnancy?

Yes, many antacids are considered safe during pregnancy. However, it's crucial to choose the right ones and use them appropriately. Avoid antacids that contain high levels of sodium or those with aluminium, as these can have adverse effects. Always consult your healthcare provider before starting any medication to ensure it's safe for you and your baby.

Are there any natural remedies for heartburn?

Yes, there are several natural remedies that can help alleviate heartburn. These include dietary adjustments, lifestyle changes, and herbal remedies. For instance, ginger, chamomile tea, and chewing gum can sometimes provide relief. We'll explore these in detail in the following sections.

Will heartburn continue after I give birth?

For most women, heartburn improves significantly after giving birth. The hormonal changes and the physical pressure from the baby that contribute to heartburn are no longer factors once your pregnancy is over. However, if you continue to experience heartburn, it's a good idea to consult your healthcare provider to rule out other potential causes.

Quick Tips for Immediate Relief

When heartburn strikes, you need fast and effective relief. Here are some quick tips that can help alleviate symptoms almost immediately.

Elevate Your Upper Body

If you're experiencing heartburn, especially at night, try elevating your upper body. Propping yourself up with pillows or using a wedge pillow can help prevent stomach acid from rising up into your esophagus. This simple adjustment can make a significant difference.

Chew Gum

Chewing gum stimulates saliva production, which can help neutralize stomach acid and wash it back down into your stomach. Opt for sugar-free gum to avoid unnecessary calories and potential tooth decay.

Eat Smaller, More Frequent Meals

Instead of three large meals a day, try eating smaller, more frequent meals. This can prevent your stomach from becoming too full and reduce the likelihood of acid reflux. Remember to eat slowly and chew your food thoroughly.

Sip on Ginger Tea

Ginger has natural anti-inflammatory properties and can help soothe the digestive tract. Sipping on ginger tea can provide quick relief from heartburn symptoms. You can make ginger tea by steeping fresh ginger slices in hot water or using ginger tea bags.

Avoid Trigger Foods

Certain foods are known to trigger heartburn. Common culprits include spicy foods, fatty foods, chocolate, caffeine, and citrus fruits. Identifying and avoiding your personal trigger foods can provide immediate relief and prevent future episodes.

Stay Upright After Eating

After meals, try to stay upright for at least an hour. Sitting or standing helps keep stomach acid where it belongs. Avoid lying down or reclining immediately after eating, as this can encourage acid to flow back into the oesophagus.

Drink Almond Milk

Almond milk is alkaline and can help neutralise stomach acid. Drinking a small glass of almond milk can provide quick relief. Additionally, almond milk is a good source of calcium and can be a healthy addition to your diet.

Try Over-the-Counter Antacids

If natural remedies aren't providing enough relief, over-the-counter antacids can be very effective. Products containing calcium carbonate, such as Tums or Rolaids, can neutralise stomach acid quickly. Be sure to follow the dosage instructions and consult with your healthcare provider if you have any concerns.

Long-Term Management Strategies

While quick fixes are great for immediate relief, managing heartburn in the long term requires a more comprehensive approach. Here are some strategies to help you keep heartburn at bay throughout your pregnancy.

Maintain a Healthy Diet

A balanced diet is crucial for managing heartburn. Focus on eating nutrient-dense foods that are easy to digest. Incorporate plenty of vegetables, lean proteins, and whole grains into your meals. Avoid foods that are high in fat, spicy, or acidic, as these can trigger heartburn.

Stay Hydrated

Drinking plenty of water throughout the day can help dilute stomach acid and reduce the risk of heartburn. However, avoid drinking large amounts of water with meals, as this can increase stomach pressure and lead to reflux. Aim to drink small sips of water between meals instead.

Wear Loose-Fitting Clothing

Tight clothing can put additional pressure on your stomach, exacerbating heartburn symptoms. Opt for loose-fitting, comfortable clothes, especially around your abdomen. Maternity wear is designed to be both stylish and comfortable, providing the support you need without added pressure.

Practice Mindful Eating

Mindful eating involves paying attention to the flavours, textures, and sensations of your food. Eating slowly and savouring each bite can help you recognize when you're full and prevent overeating. This practice can also reduce stress, which can be a trigger for heartburn.

Incorporate Gentle Exercise

Regular physical activity can help improve digestion and reduce the risk of heartburn. Activities such as walking, swimming, and prenatal yoga are excellent choices. Avoid vigorous exercise immediately after eating, as this can worsen symptoms. Instead, opt for gentle activities that promote relaxation and well-being.

Monitor Your Weight Gain

While weight gain is a normal and healthy part of pregnancy, excessive weight gain can increase the risk of heartburn. Work with your healthcare provider to ensure you're gaining weight at a healthy rate. They can provide guidance on nutrition and exercise to support your overall health.

Consider Sleeping on Your Left Side

Sleeping on your left side can help reduce the risk of heartburn. This position keeps your stomach below your oesophagus, making it less likely for acid to flow back up. Using a pregnancy pillow can provide additional support and comfort, helping you maintain this position throughout the night.

Practice Relaxation Techniques

Stress can be a major trigger for heartburn. Incorporate relaxation techniques into your daily routine to help manage stress. Deep breathing exercises, meditation, and prenatal massage can all be effective ways to promote relaxation and reduce stress levels.

Keep a Food Diary

Keeping a food diary can help you identify patterns and triggers for your heartburn. Record what you eat, when you eat, and any symptoms you experience. Over time, you'll be able to pinpoint specific foods or habits that contribute to your heartburn and make informed adjustments.

Consult with a Healthcare Provider

Regular check-ins with your healthcare provider are essential for managing heartburn during pregnancy. They can provide personalised advice, monitor your progress, and adjust your treatment plan as needed. Don't hesitate to reach out if you have any concerns or if your symptoms persist despite your best efforts.

By following these long-term management strategies, you can significantly reduce the frequency and severity of heartburn episodes. Remember, every pregnancy is unique, and what works for one person may not work for another. Be patient with yourself and open to trying different approaches until you find what works best for you. With the right strategies and support, you can manage heartburn effectively and enjoy a more comfortable and healthy pregnancy.

CONCLUSION

As we reach the conclusion of our journey together, I want to take a moment to reflect on the essential insights and practical advice we've explored. Managing heartburn during pregnancy is not just about alleviating discomfort; it's about enhancing your overall well-being and ensuring a smoother, more enjoyable pregnancy experience. Throughout this book, we've delved into the causes and symptoms of heartburn, the critical role of diet and lifestyle, safe medications and treatments, holistic approaches, and much more. Each chapter has been designed to provide you with a comprehensive understanding and actionable strategies to manage heartburn effectively.

One of the fundamental takeaways is the importance of understanding why heartburn occurs during pregnancy. By recognizing the hormonal and physical changes your body undergoes, you can better appreciate why heartburn is such a common issue. Hormones like progesterone play a vital role in relaxing the muscles of your uterus, but they also relax the valve between your esophagus and stomach, leading to acid reflux. Additionally, as your baby grows, the increased pressure on your stomach can exacerbate heartburn. Understanding these mechanisms is the first step toward managing the symptoms.

Dietary changes are a cornerstone of heartburn management. We've discussed how certain foods and beverages can trigger heartburn, while others can help soothe your digestive system. By avoiding trigger foods like spicy dishes, citrus fruits, and caffeine, and incorporating heartburn-friendly options like oatmeal, ginger, and yogurt, you can significantly reduce the frequency and severity of heartburn episodes. Meal planning and mindful eating habits, such as eating smaller, more frequent meals and avoiding late-night snacks, are simple yet effective strategies to keep heartburn at bay.

Lifestyle modifications also play a crucial role. Adjusting your sleeping position, for instance, by elevating the head of your bed or using pillows to keep your upper body slightly upright, can prevent stomach acid from flowing back into your esophagus. Stress management techniques, such as practicing yoga, meditation, or simply taking time to relax and unwind, are essential. Stress can exacerbate heartburn, so finding ways to stay calm and centered is vital for your overall well-being.

When it comes to medications and treatments, safety is paramount. We've reviewed over-the-counter remedies, prescription medications, and natural supplements that can provide relief without posing a risk to you or your baby. Always consult with your healthcare provider before starting any new treatment to ensure it aligns with your specific needs and circumstances.

Holistic and alternative approaches offer additional avenues for relief. Herbal remedies, acupuncture, and gentle exercise like prenatal yoga can complement conventional treatments and provide a more comprehensive approach to managing heartburn. These methods can be particularly beneficial if you're looking to minimise medication use or if you prefer a more natural approach.

Dealing with severe heartburn requires vigilance and proactive measures. Recognizing the signs of severe heartburn and knowing when to seek medical intervention is crucial. Persistent heartburn can lead to complications such as esophagitis, so it's important to address severe cases promptly and effectively. Your healthcare provider can offer targeted treatments and support to manage severe symptoms and ensure your health and comfort.

Throughout this book, personal stories and experiences have illustrated the challenges and triumphs of managing heartburn during pregnancy. Hearing from other mothers and healthcare professionals provides valuable perspectives and practical tips that you can apply to your own situation. These stories remind us that you're not alone in this journey, and there are effective solutions and supportive communities available to help you.

As we conclude, I want to leave you with some final thoughts and encouragement. Pregnancy is a unique and transformative time in your life, filled with anticipation, joy, and sometimes a few challenges. Heartburn may be one of those challenges, but with the knowledge and strategies you've gained from this book, you're well-equipped to manage it effectively. Remember that every pregnancy is different, and what works for one person may not work for another. Be patient with yourself as you find the best approaches for your body and your lifestyle.

It's also important to stay connected with your healthcare provider. Regular check-ups and open communication with your doctor are essential for monitoring your health and addressing any concerns that arise. Don't hesitate to seek medical advice if you're struggling with severe or persistent heartburn. Your doctor can provide personalized guidance and support to ensure you and your baby stay healthy and comfortable.

Moving forward with confidence is key. You've learned about the causes and symptoms of heartburn, dietary and lifestyle changes that can make a difference, safe medications and treatments, holistic approaches, and how to handle severe cases.

Armed with this knowledge, you can make informed decisions and take proactive steps to manage heartburn and enjoy a more comfortable pregnancy.

Remember to take care of yourself, both physically and emotionally. Pregnancy is a time of significant change, and it's important to prioritise self-care. Whether it's through nourishing meals, gentle exercise, relaxation techniques, or simply taking time for yourself, these practices will support your overall well-being and help you manage heartburn more effectively.

As you look ahead to the arrival of your baby, focus on the joy and excitement of this special time. Managing heartburn is just one aspect of your pregnancy journey, and with the right strategies, you can minimise its impact and concentrate on the positive moments. Celebrate the milestones, cherish the small victories, and embrace the journey ahead with confidence and optimism.

Thank you for allowing me to be a part of your pregnancy journey. I hope this book has provided you with valuable insights, practical advice, and the reassurance that you can manage heartburn effectively. Remember, you're not alone, and there are resources and support available to help you every step of the way. Here's to a healthy, happy, and heartburn-free pregnancy!

GLOSSARY OF TERMS

As you navigate this journey of managing heartburn during pregnancy, you'll come across a variety of terms and concepts that may be new to you. To make this journey smoother and more comprehensible, I've compiled a glossary of key terms that you'll encounter throughout this book. This section is designed to be a quick reference guide, providing clear and concise definitions to help you understand and apply the information effectively.

Acid Reflux: A condition where stomach acid flows back into the oesophagus, causing irritation and a burning sensation, commonly referred to as heartburn.

Antacids: Medications that neutralise stomach acid to relieve heartburn and indigestion. They are available over-the-counter and are often used for quick relief.

Bile Reflux: A condition where bile, a digestive fluid produced by the liver, backs up into the stomach and esophagus, causing irritation similar to acid reflux.

Diaphragm: A large, dome-shaped muscle located at the base of the lungs that plays a key role in breathing. Its contraction helps increase the pressure in the abdomen, which can affect heartburn symptoms.

Esophagitis: Inflammation of the oesophagus, often caused by acid reflux. Symptoms include pain, difficulty swallowing, and a burning sensation.

Gastroesophageal Reflux Disease (GERD): A chronic condition where acid reflux occurs more than twice a week, causing persistent symptoms and potential damage to the oesophagus.

Hiatal Hernia: A condition where part of the stomach pushes up through the diaphragm into the chest cavity, often exacerbating heartburn and acid reflux.

Lower Esophageal Sphincter (LES): A ring of muscle at the bottom of the oesophagus that acts as a valve, preventing stomach acid from flowing back into the oesophagus. During pregnancy, hormonal changes can relax this muscle, leading to heartburn.

pH Levels: A measure of how acidic or basic a substance is. The stomach typically has a low pH (high acidity) to aid in digestion, but this can contribute to heartburn if acid reflux occurs.

Progesterone: A hormone that increases during pregnancy to help maintain the pregnancy. It also relaxes the muscles in the digestive tract, including the LES, which can lead to increased heartburn.

Proton Pump Inhibitors (PPIs): Medications that reduce the production of stomach acid, providing longer-lasting relief from heartburn and acid reflux. They are often prescribed for severe or chronic cases.

Reflux: The backward flow of stomach acid or bile into the oesophagus, leading to symptoms such as heartburn, regurgitation, and irritation of the oesophagus.

Trimesters: The three stages of pregnancy, each lasting about three months. Heartburn can vary in intensity and frequency throughout the different trimesters.

Understanding these terms will empower you to better grasp the concepts discussed in this book and communicate more effectively with your healthcare provider. As you encounter these terms, refer back to this glossary for a quick refresher.

Dietary Charts and Meal Plans

Managing heartburn during pregnancy often involves making thoughtful dietary choices. Certain foods can trigger heartburn, while others can help alleviate symptoms. In this section, I've put together dietary charts and meal plans designed to provide you with delicious, nutritious options that minimise heartburn and support your overall health.

Foods to Avoid:

1. Spicy Foods: Spices like chili powder, black pepper, and hot peppers can irritate the oesophagus and increase heartburn.
2. Citrus Fruits: Oranges, lemons, limes, and grapefruits are highly acidic and can exacerbate heartburn.
3. Tomato-Based Products: Tomatoes and tomato sauces are acidic and can trigger heartburn.

4. Caffeinated Beverages: Coffee, tea, and soda can relax the LES and stimulate stomach acid production.
5. Fried and Fatty Foods: High-fat foods can slow down digestion and increase the risk of reflux.
6. Chocolate: Contains both caffeine and fat, which can trigger heartburn.
7. Carbonated Drinks: Carbonation can cause bloating and increase pressure on the LES.

Heartburn-Friendly Foods:

1. Non-Citrus Fruits: Bananas, melons, apples, and pears are less likely to trigger heartburn.
2. Vegetables: Leafy greens, broccoli, cauliflower, carrots, and green beans are low in acid and beneficial for digestion.
3. Lean Proteins: Chicken, turkey, fish, and tofu are easier on the stomach compared to high-fat meats.

4. Whole Grains: Oatmeal, brown rice, whole-wheat bread, and quinoa provide fibre and aid digestion.

5. Low-Fat Dairy: Skim milk, yogurt, and low-fat cheese are less likely to cause heartburn.

6. Ginger: Known for its anti-inflammatory properties, ginger can help soothe the digestive tract.

7. Herbal Teas: Chamomile and ginger tea can be calming and reduce heartburn symptoms.

Sample Meal Plan:

Breakfast:
- Oatmeal topped with sliced bananas and a drizzle of honey.
- Herbal tea (chamomile or ginger).

Mid-Morning Snack:
- A handful of almonds and an apple.

Lunch:

- Grilled chicken salad with mixed greens, cucumbers, carrots, and a light vinaigrette dressing.
- Whole-wheat bread.

Afternoon Snack:
- Greek yoghourt with a sprinkle of granola.

Dinner:
- Baked salmon with a side of steamed broccoli and quinoa.
- Melon slices for dessert.

Evening Snack:
- A small bowl of sliced melon or a handful of baby carrots.

This meal plan is designed to provide balanced nutrition while minimising heartburn triggers. Feel free to mix and match the foods listed to create meals that suit your taste and nutritional needs.

Sample Exercises and Yoga Poses

Regular physical activity can play a significant role in managing heartburn during pregnancy. Gentle exercises and yoga poses can help improve digestion, reduce stress, and promote overall well-being. In this section, I'll share some safe and effective exercises and yoga poses that are particularly beneficial for pregnant women experiencing heartburn.

Gentle Exercises:

1. Walking: A simple and effective way to stay active without putting too much strain on your body. Aim for a 30-minute walk daily, ideally after meals to aid digestion.
2. Swimming: Provides a full-body workout while reducing stress on your joints. Swimming can help improve circulation and digestion.
3. Pelvic Tilts: Stand with your back against a wall, knees slightly bent. Tilt your pelvis forward and hold for a few seconds, then

release. Repeat 10-15 times. This exercise can help alleviate back pain and improve posture.

4. Prenatal Pilates: Focuses on strengthening the core muscles, improving posture, and enhancing flexibility. Look for classes or online videos specifically designed for pregnant women.

Yoga Poses:

1. Cat-Cow Pose (Marjaryasana-Bitilasana):
  - Start on your hands and knees, with your wrists directly under your shoulders and your knees under your hips.
  - Inhale and arch your back, lifting your head and tailbone towards the ceiling (Cow Pose).
  - Exhale and round your back, tucking your chin to your chest and drawing your belly button towards your spine (Cat Pose).
  - Repeat for 10-15 breaths, moving slowly and gently.

2. Child's Pose (Balasana):

- Kneel on the floor with your big toes touching and knees spread wide apart.
- Sit back on your heels and extend your arms forward, lowering your torso to the floor.
- Rest your forehead on the mat and take deep breaths, holding the pose for 1-2 minutes.
- This pose helps relieve tension in the back and neck, promoting relaxation.

3. Seated Forward Bend (Paschimottanasana):

- Sit on the floor with your legs extended straight in front of you.
- Inhale and lengthen your spine, reaching your arms overhead.
- Exhale and hinge at your hips, reaching towards your toes while keeping your spine straight.

- Hold the pose for 1-2 minutes, focusing on your breath.
- This pose can help improve digestion and relieve tension in the lower back.

4. Supported Bridge Pose (Setu Bandhasana):

- Lie on your back with your knees bent and feet hip-width apart, flat on the floor.
- Place a yoga block or firm cushion under your sacrum for support.
- Lift your hips and rest them on the block, allowing your back to relax.
- Hold the pose for 1-2 minutes, breathing deeply.
- This pose can help alleviate lower back pain and improve circulation.

5. Reclining Bound Angle Pose (Supta Baddha Konasana):

- Lie on your back with your knees bent and the soles of your feet together.

- Allow your knees to drop open, creating a gentle stretch in your inner thighs.
   - Place pillows or cushions under your knees for support if needed.
   - Rest your hands on your belly and focus on deep, calming breaths.
   - Hold the pose for 1-2 minutes, promoting relaxation and reducing stress.

These exercises and yoga poses are designed to be gentle and safe for pregnant women. Always listen to your body and avoid any movements that cause discomfort. If you're new to exercise or yoga, consider consulting with a prenatal fitness instructor or your healthcare provider before starting a new routine.

By incorporating these exercises and yoga poses into your daily routine, you can improve your overall well-being and better manage heartburn during pregnancy. Remember, staying active and taking time for yourself are essential components of a healthy, balanced pregnancy.

As you continue your journey through pregnancy, it's essential to focus on your well-being, both physically and mentally. The exercises and yoga poses suggested in this book are not only intended to help manage heartburn but also to enhance your overall health and bring a sense of calm and relaxation to your daily routine. Taking time for yourself each day, even if it's just a few minutes of stretching or a short walk, can make a significant difference in how you feel.

Incorporating these practices into your lifestyle can also foster a deeper connection with your body and your baby. Mindful movement, such as yoga, encourages you to tune into your breath and be present in the moment, which can be incredibly grounding during the often overwhelming experience of pregnancy. This mindfulness can help reduce stress and anxiety, making it easier to handle the physical and emotional changes you're going through.

When it comes to exercise, it's crucial to prioritize safety and listen to your body. Pregnancy is not the time to push your limits or try new, strenuous activities. Instead, focus on gentle, consistent movement that feels good and supports your overall health. Remember to stay hydrated, wear comfortable clothing, and avoid exercising in extreme heat.

If you're new to yoga or exercise, consider joining a prenatal class or seeking guidance from a certified prenatal instructor. These professionals can provide personalized advice and modifications to ensure that your practice is safe and effective. Additionally, prenatal classes offer a wonderful opportunity to connect with other expectant mothers, creating a supportive community where you can share experiences and advice.

In summary, the exercises and yoga poses provided in this book are designed to be a safe and effective way to manage heartburn and promote overall well-being during pregnancy. By incorporating these practices into your routine, you can improve your digestion, reduce stress, and foster a deeper connection with your body and your baby. Remember to listen to your body, prioritize safety, and enjoy the journey.

The Appendices section of this book is intended to be a practical resource, offering tools and information that you can refer to throughout your pregnancy. The glossary of terms provides clear definitions to help you understand the concepts discussed in the book. The dietary charts and meal plans offer practical guidance on making healthy food choices that minimize heartburn, while the sample exercises and yoga poses provide a gentle, effective way to stay active and manage stress.

As you embark on this journey, remember that you are not alone. Heartburn is a common experience during pregnancy, and with the right knowledge and strategies, you can manage it effectively. This book is here to support you every step of the way, providing you with the tools and information you need to enjoy a healthy, comfortable pregnancy.

Thank you for allowing me to be a part of your journey. I hope that the information and insights shared in this book help you feel empowered and confident as you navigate the challenges and joys of pregnancy. May your journey be filled with health, happiness, and heartburn-free days.